THE CALL

A daughter's journey down
the road of Dementia with her mother

Magda L. Walker

The Call
© May 2017 Magda L. Walker All Rights Reserved
Published May 2017 by Magda L. Walker

ISBN: 978-0-9988048-0-4

Contact the publisher and/or author at:
Walk3Roads@aol.com

Credits:

Cover Art: shutterstock Stock photo ID: 99385142

Layout, Editing and Book Design: Alane Pearce of Alane Pearce Professional Writing Services LLC. Learn more at MyPublishingCoach.com

Publishing coaching, and project management by Alane Pearce, Professional Writing Services, LLC. Contact at MyPublishingCoach.com or email at alane@MyPublishingCoach.com

Walker, Magda L.: The Call

1. Memoir   2. Adult Care   3. Dementia

ACKNOWLEDGMENTS

I would like to say thank you to Ingham County Medical Care Facility in Okemos, Michigan. To every single staff from Admitting to her Doctors and Nurses and Aides; I cannot thank you enough for your help and kindness. Not only did you help my Mother with her transition but mine as well. You are truly are called to do what you do. The patience and love you showed my Mother will always be appreciated.

First I would like to thank my husband of 31 years, Fred for your love and support.

Uncle Fred, thank you for being there for mom all those years after dad died. God bless you.

My cousins, Rosie and Wesley Vargas from Minnesota who never got tired of listening to me vent, who offered me spiritual advice and prayer.

To my "Primas," Elida, Ofelia, Robin and Liz.

To my daughters; Elisa Quintero, Lena Bailey and Tasha Walker who helped me with mother.

I would also like to thank my son, Freddie Walker, for his support and keeping me in prayer.

Special thanks to my best friend, Donna Peace, for her help and encouragement to write my story.

Mary Barnes, I thank you for reading my book and inspiring me to publish. You were instrumental in the completion of my book.

And last but not least, Nurse Liz Quintero, who is also my cousin. Thank you.

The Ugly Beast Named Dementia

I never ran so fast in my life like the night I got the call. The Nurse said, "Laty, I think your mom has taken a turn for the worse. You better come in."

I said, "I am on my way."

The nurse was waiting for me and the night entrance door. She quickly opened the door and just said, "Hurry."

I ran to my mom's corridor. Her room was all the way at the end. I went in her room, dropped my purse on the floor. I ran to her and leaned over the bed and looked at her. Her eyes were open, but in a stare. She could not speak anymore but they tell me that the hearing is the last to go. I said to her, "Mom, I am here. It's okay, you can go."

And then her last breath.

I am writing my story about my life with a parent with dementia in the hopes of shedding light on this disease from a personal perspective. As more and more baby boomers are faced with caring for their elderly parents,

I wanted to share my experience.

My story is not one of a wonderful mother/daughter relationship. She was not my best friend. She also was not my enemy. I loved my mother and feel she loved me. We had our problems but it never stopped us from being family.

I spoke with my mother almost every day. Sometimes just to say good morning or good night, and sometimes to talk for hours. I did try to honor my parents, especially in their later years. My mother was a strict disciplinarian and didn't like to joke around. She was a great cook and very clean and kept her children presentable always. She was a very faithful and loyal wife to my father. For that I am grateful.

In her later years when the dementia started it was extremely hard to face the change in her, like the harsh words that would come out of her mouth. Even though you tell yourself they can't help it, if feels like they mean every word and it cuts like a knife. If you are facing this in your life, know that they do not have control or filters that are normally in place and try not to take it personally. Let love for your parents get you through this very trying time. You will get through this. I did. With the help of almighty God and the beautiful people He put in my life to help me in my journey, I made it and you will too.

The Journey Begins

I remember how our journey started with this ugly beast named dementia. I know it is an illness, but it is awful. To have your body but not your mind is horrible. I think it is harder for the family and friends of a dementia patient to accept the diagnosis and live with it. The patient doesn't see it or know they have it.

When I first tried to tell my mother she had dementia she would say, "But I don't feel anything. I don't feel sick." The most I remember is she would catch herself making mistakes, or forgetting things and trying to cover up with excuses. She would get frustrated when she realized she had done something twice because she did not remember doing it the first time. Or if you brought to her attention that she had already asked a question and she didn't remember asking she would get upset.

There were times when she just seemed far away. She was in her own thoughts. She lost interest in her favorite television shows because she couldn't remember the story lines or even the actors. When others were talking she seemed uninterested in the conversation. Those were the subtle ways the disease began to manifest. It would progress as time went on. The tears run down my face as I remember how it all started for us, when I lost my mother the first time.

Her Life

My mother, Maria, was a very strong willed and strong-minded person. She had a very deep faith in her Catholicism and the Virgin Mary. She was an extremely hard-working woman. She was a stay at home mom and took great pride in keeping a very clean house. No one cooked better Mexican food than my mom. She was an excellent cook. When my father came home from work, his dinner was always ready. They don't make housewives like that anymore. She was old school for sure but she was not a weak woman. My father ruled the roost but mother was not shy in voicing her opinions. If she had been given an opportunity to go to school past the second grade, she would have been a force to be reckoned with. She was very smart, had good common sense and was well mannered. My parents were married in 1947. She was 21 years old. Their marriage would last 59 years until my father died.

My father was from Mexico and my mother was from Texas. They met on the international bridge crossing from Nuevo Laredo, Mexico to Laredo, Texas. She had to cross the bridge every day to go to work on the

Mexican side. My father would see her walking and follow her after work on her way back across the bridge to the American side. He would follow up to the point of where they collected the toll for using the bridge, at that time it was ten cents. Finally, one day she asked him, hey why don't you follow me across to the other side? He replied, because I do not have the ten cents to pay! That was their cute love story they liked to remember. Of course, he finally did get a job and have enough not only to follow her across the bridge, but enough to ask for her hand in marriage. Her father said yes. Her mother had passed when she was still a girl.

By the time she met my father, her siblings were all grown and most were married or in the service. She was raised by a few different stepmothers as my grandpa remarried a few times. They were not very nice to her but she understood her father needed a woman to take care of him. I think that is why mom was so tough. She never let anyone hurt her again. She had a hard young life.

She and my father dated for one year and then they were married. They lived in Texas for a few years and moved to Michigan before I was born. I had two brothers born before me, one in Mexico and the other in Michigan in the 1950's. Mom had a sister in Michigan so they moved there looking for a better life for us. Dad took a variety of jobs from construction to working in a steel foundry. He would eventually get a job with GM at the Fisher Body plant in Lansing, MI. They would remain in Lansing for the rest of their marriage. Dad retired from Fisher Body in 1991. Mother was always a stay at home mom. They had a nice home and always had a nice car. We went to Catholic school at a great sacrifice. But it is what my parents wanted for us, as they did not finish school. My mother did attend adult education when I was a teenager.

Although my mother could speak English well and was able to converse with the teachers and the neighbors, her reading and writing was limited. I complained to her that my friend's mothers could drive and take them to school and sporting events and she could not take me. So she signed up for driving courses and got her driver's license at the age of 44. She loved school; it was good for her.

Because she spoke two languages, we were raised bilingual, Spanish and English. I was able to translate at a very young age. Often I would accompany my father to the bank and translate for him if he had trouble understanding something. It was great for us children as it helped us in the long run.

My father would become an American citizen when my oldest brother was only 7 years old. And my brother also became an American citizen and would grow up to serve in the Viet Nam war. We all cried the day the Army took him to Nam and it was the longest year of our lives, but he made it back by the grace of God. The year he was gone my mother lit a candle every day as a promise to God for the return of her son.

By the time Jerry, my oldest brother, came home my other brother, Rey Jr., had graduated from high school and I was in high school. We all graduated from high school and that made my parents very happy.

My dad's cousin, Alfredo Martinez, came to live with us just after I was born. We grew up with him as an older brother/uncle. He served in the Marine Corps and moved to Michigan to seek a better life. He was single and remained so during our life together with my parents. Uncle Fred is a big part of my story, as you will see.

As all of us children grew and left the nest, Uncle Fred remained with them for the rest of their lives. He never married, as he was the sole provider for his parents in Texas. They lived very long, blessed lives, but by the time they passed Uncle Fred felt he was too old to get married. He was past being able to have children of his own and took us and the other children of the family in as his own. He also took care of my mom and dad in their silver years. They were in pretty good shape into their 70's. Dad just didn't care to do the lawn care of the house and outside work. Uncle Fred loved it so it worked out for them. They shared the expenses and it was a good arrangement, until my father became ill.

Life after Dad

My father was a very healthy man. Never took any kind of medicine. Great vision too! He was a good-looking, green-eyed, handsome man. One day, he complained about a fungal issue with his feet. By now he was in his late 70's. The doctor prescribed an oral anti-fungal medicine with a side effect of damaging the kidneys if taken more than twice. Well, it did indeed cause his kidneys to fail and he started dialysis the following year of taking that medication.

He was such an amazing man. He never complained about his plight. He did what he had to do to survive. However, the food and salt and water restrictions put on him made him lose 40 lbs. the first year. He got weak and had to stop driving. He left more and more responsibilities for Uncle Fred. After another year of becoming more and more frail, he could no longer do his share of the work. He tried to do all the doctors told him to do and tried to limit his coffee and water. It was very hard, but he fought the good fight. He lasted two years with kidney failure until he suffered a heart attack. It did not kill him instantly. He was rushed to the hospital where he was told he had a heart attack and there was nothing they could do for him.

It was a beautiful last day for him. He was able to speak and say his good byes to his loved ones. He even got to see my daughter who flew in from California to be married the next weekend. She made it to the hospital running, literally, but was able to tell him good-bye. He also met with his priest for his last prayers. He was surrounded with family and love.

He asked my Uncle Fred if he would remain in the house where they were all living and to take care of Maria. Of course, he said yes he would take care of her. Dad passed that same night, peacefully knowing mom would be well taken care of. He was 82.

Now life would begin for Uncle Fred and my mother. They knew each other's ways and got along well after living together for so many years. They hardest part was just missing dad. Uncle Fred was retired and used to the routine of the chores and meals. He was such a big help to my mother. She could not have remained in her home without him. She was full of arthritis in her hands and needed quite a bit of assistance with the cooking and the chores. She wanted to remain independent and did not want to live with her kids. By this time my middle brother Rey had passed. He was only 40. That left my oldest brother and myself to help Uncle Fred with Mom.

I lived 90 miles away and only came to town once a week. I would bring meals and help with the cleaning and give Uncle Fred a break. He was, after all, with my mom 24/7. The good thing is they enjoyed the same programs on TV and she liked his cooking. Everything pretty much remained the same as life was before dad passed.

The First Signs

The first couple of years seemed to go on without incident. I mean there was the usual forgetfulness you'd expect from someone who is eighty. For instance, Mom would say, "Why haven't you called?" And I would say, "Mom, I called you this morning, remember we talked about me coming over?"

"No, no you haven't called."

Then she would get upset as if you were lying. Then she started forgetting where she put things, like her money. I would ask her why didn't she just put her money in her purse and she would say it was because she had to put it somewhere safe. Well I didn't understand that at first because Uncle Fred and I were the only ones in the house with her. He had never taken anything of hers and neither had I.

It happened because she couldn't remember where she hid her money. She would spend hours looking for it, sometimes she would find it and other times not. I asked her to quit hiding her money. I didn't think that was anything to worry about, I just thought it was old age. What I would learn later was that it was paranoia from the dementia and her short-term memory starting to fail.

Since Uncle Fred was in charge of the meals, he started to notice Mom becoming more bothered by his attempt to not feed her too much. Mother had a weight issue most of her silver years and was quite heavy for a little lady of her height. So, Uncle Fred would try not to put too much food on her plate, but she would get mad if you suggested she was eating too much. She started demanding that he put dishes of food on the table so she could serve herself. Her excuse was she liked to eat well at noon and a light dinner. But what she ate at noon was enough for both meals. This was going to become an issue they did not have before. She was weighing over 200 lbs. for her 5' frame. If he would tell her to cut down on her portions, she would start getting mad and she would tell him or anyone else, to leave her alone. Uncle Fred did not like to argue with her so he stopped saying anything to her about it.

This was a little different behavior than he was used to. And although we noticed she was acting out more, we just thought that Mom was getting a little touchy in her old age. One other factor I always believed had something to do with her mood swings was the fact that she stopped taking a female hormone after 40 some years. Somehow, this prescription slipped through the cracks of her health care physicians. It was initially prescribed when she had a hysterectomy at 40. When I took over her health care and was taking her to the doctor I asked why she was still on this hormone and they said she should not have been taking it so they removed her from it. This drug is advertised on TV as possible dementia as a side effect. I don't know if that contributed to Mother's dementia or not but it is possible.

Those were some of the first signs Uncle Fred noticed from day-to-day living that were changing.

Uncle Fred Goes on Vacation

The first year Uncle Fred took care of Mom by himself after Dad's passing, I came to stay with Mother so he could take a vacation. He would go to Texas to visit his two brothers and their families. My mother did not like when I came to stay with her and let Uncle Fred go. She was very possessive of him. He was her caregiver. She became very attached to him. He spoiled her, just like my dad did. But what we didn't know is that when you have dementia, you do not like change. Because I did things a little different than Uncle Fred, she complained and was unhappy. I thought it was just me she didn't like. She was almost mean to me. She was always bossy, but now it seemed to be getting worse because she would get angry. We had known she was suffering with dementia at this point. This is the first time I would stay with my mother for an extended length of time 24/7. This gave me a real indication of what Uncle Fred was dealing with.

One day while I was there one of her friends, actually, a shirt-tail relative, came over with some food for her. She often stayed to visit and eat lunch with mom and Uncle Fred. When I cooked I would invite her over too as

I appreciated what she did for my mom and Uncle Fred. We were sitting eating lunch and when we were done, I offered our guest to take some food home as we had far too much. I was shocked that my mother responded quickly that she was not going to take any food home. My mother said, "She has food at home, she doesn't need to take mine!"

My mother never reacted like that before. She was always generous when it came to food and gave food away as a kind gesture. So this was not like her at all. Of course, the lady said, "It's fine; I do have food at home I don't need to take any."

I thought about what happened and wondered if mom was having flashbacks to her childhood. That may have been the only time she did not have plenty to eat. They were poor and didn't have much. You did not throw food away and you ate everything on your plate and you did not waste anything. Another sign, that we would recognize after her diagnosis, of the start of dementia.

I don't know all the clinical reasons the long-term memory is present more than the short-term memory as you age, but more and more we were seeing her live in the past. She would talk about things that happened 60 years ago as if it were yesterday. Like she would tell people that she was going to go see her cousin who was a doctor, (who by the way was in another state, Texas) because the doctors I was taking her to here in Michigan did not know what they were talking about. She started talking like she could take care of herself and she could get to the doctor on her own, when in reality she could not. There was a doctor in the family some 40 years ago on my dad's side of the family, but mother had never seen him as a physician. I didn't know why she was bringing him up now. What I learned about dementia is that you cannot reason with someone who is unreasonable. My mother could no longer reason.

I was having difficulty convincing her she did not have to hoard food, or clothes for that matter. She had every closet in the house full of her old clothes that she would not let me get rid of. She had the same issue with money, not wanting to spend any money. The paranoia was setting in.

One more story that happened on my watch while Uncle Fred was on vacation was the "blouse" situation. I will never forget that she asked me to get a blouse that was hanging on the back of the bathroom door. We were seated in the living room with my two cousins who had come to visit. One of the cousins is Nurse Liz, who would become my lifeline. I went to the bathroom to get the blouse and it was not there. I came back out into the living room where she was seated and told her it was not there, asking if she could have put it somewhere else. She got very defensive and said it was there and she knew where she left it. She got so angry with me and actually accused me of lying. If my cousins weren't there to witness this behavior, I don't think anyone would have believed me. She said I was trying to make her go crazy and I wasn't telling the truth. She was raising her voice and getting quite upset with me. I said, "MOM, slow down, you probably just forgot where you put it!"

At this point, I was still thinking this was normal old age forgetfulness. I did finally find the blouse when I opened the basement door and saw it was on the steps as if someone threw it down to be washed. They did that sometimes. Instead of walking all the way down to the laundry room, they would toss it down the stairs and pick it up later. I was so happy to tell her I found it so she wouldn't wonder about it. I explained to her that she must have thrown it downstairs and forgot. The fury she unleashed on me was unimaginable. She screamed at me and said I must have thrown it down there and I was lying!

I said, "I did not throw it down there Mom, why would I lie to you?" Well that just made her angrier and I did not understand at that moment what was happening.

My cousin, Nurse Liz, quickly stepped in and redirected the conversation and got her to calm down. Nurse Liz is a geriatric nurse and has much experience with the elderly. I just looked at my cousins and they looked at me and we all wondered what just happened. We spoke of the blouse no more.

Night Time

I slept in the room next to hers at night so I could hear her when she got up to use the bathroom. She could still walk but with a walker. She had fallen a few times so we were more vigilant at nighttime. Mother would blame her falls on her knees. She thought something was wrong with her replacements, as both her knees had been replaced. What was happening is she was shuffling her feet instead of picking them up. I thought that was normal for a gal her age. It was easy to trip on a rug or corner of a piece of furniture you know. She would get up sometimes three times a night. I didn't get much sleep as a result of waking with her every couple of hours. I would make sure she got back in bed, and then I could go back to bed too. I understood why Uncle Fred was taking naps during the day because he was probably getting up with her too, or at least hearing her move about.

In the morning I made her coffee and breakfast for her just like Uncle Fred did, as mother couldn't get around the kitchen anymore. She had a routine. She took her medicines and checked her sugar. After breakfast she would get cleaned up for the day. Washed her face and brushed her teeth so she was ready for the rest of the day.

She would go sit in the living room to watch her shows until lunch. Then lunch had to be prepared and served for her. Clean up after lunch. Then she would take a nap. She would wake and ask for a magazine sometimes or talk on the phone. Then it was dinner time and again the preparation of the meal and serving and cleaning up. It occurred to me that this was what Uncle Fred was doing every day. Not to mention the laundry and daily housework. It was starting to be more than he could handle.

Memory

My mother loved to talk. Of course her stories were more and more about the past as I mentioned earlier. She started talking about me when I was a teenager. The things she brought up were as if they just happened. One of the things she remembered with such emotion was when I ran away from home. I was only 14 years old at the time. I was still a kid. In her mind, I was still mad at her and didn't "like" her. I would try and explain that it was many years ago. I never thought I was going to revisit this time of my life with her. That issue was dead and buried, so I thought. But it was funny how when made to go back to that time, all the memories come flooding back. It was crazy to me how something you have pushed way down can surface again. Like picking an old scab. It was a very painful memory for me because I loved my father so much and hated to have caused him so much pain. At the time, I didn't think my mother cared so I was not worried about her. I was gone for a week. I cannot imagine as a parent now, what I put my parents through, and the anguish of not knowing where I was or who I was with.

I came back after one week and my father was so happy. My mother looked so mad. My father asked me to sit down and tell them why I had left and she sat at the table too. I told my dad it was because of her. I did not say mother, I said her. I was very hurt and confused. My mother had let me down in a big way. That in itself is another story. It is something she and I never discussed after the fact and never did even until her death.

She was so angry at me for telling my dad it was her fault I left, that she grabbed a coffee cup on the hutch and threw it at me. I jumped up from the table and flew out the door and down the street. They couldn't catch me. I disappeared into the field that backed up to some apartments. I jumped the fence and found refuge with a friend of mine in their apartment. My family kept running down the path in the woods and did not find me. I called my brother to tell him I was all right and not to worry about me but I was not coming home. I ended up staying with a family member and they convinced me to come back home after about a week. There was so much pain in this memory for the both of us. I hated to relive it and hated that she remembered it like it was yesterday. I hated what I had put them through but at the time I did not see it. I only felt my own pain. I told her I was sorry that I had put them through that terrible ordeal, but that I was not that mixed up teenager anymore. We never brought up what led up to me running away, or ever talked about it. I chose to leave it where it was in the past. I told her I loved her and that was a long time ago and I did not feel that way now.

The second big blow to me with her memory was my divorce. She took my divorce very hard because I was the first one in my family to get a divorce. At the time I was taking care of her for Uncle Fred, I had been married to my present husband almost 30 years. It had been so long since my divorce it was inconceivable to me that after all these years she would still harbor these painful memories about it. She would bring up my divorce or mention my ex-husband almost every day. I would ask her not to mention him and I felt as if she was doing it on purpose just to pick a fight with me. I was losing my patience with her about it and hated having words with her. I did not understand. I cried so much during that stay. I did not know what I was dealing with though.

All kinds of feelings were running through my mind. If only I had known the culprit was dementia and not my mother. Sometimes I would think about what she would say like, I may be smarter than her because I finished school, but she had only been married once and to one man! She said I was ashamed of my divorce, which was not true, and I shouldn't have taken it so personally, but I did. It was so painful for me to dredge up the divorce every day with her. Something always happened and it was a direct result of my divorce she would say. I turned to drugs and alcohol to deal with my divorce.

The only reason I found my footing was God's grace and his mercy that put my feet on solid ground and helped me find my way out of the darkness. Breaking up a family and in my case involving two little girls nearly was my destruction. That is another story in itself. But I pushed on in my relationship with her. I couldn't wait for Uncle Fred to come home. I didn't know how much more I could take. The problem was she couldn't remember bringing up this painful subject with me every day. I didn't believe her at first when she would claim to not have said anything to me about my past and divorce. But she truly was not remembering.

I couldn't understand why my mom was so unhappy with me. I had been a good daughter. I cooked for them every holiday, every birthday, and on Mother's and Father's Day. I was so grateful for everything they had done for my children and me. God had given me the grace to forgive my mother for my hurtful past and to move on. I truly thought our issue was in the past to stay.

I continued to do for my mom. I loved to do hair and my mom started to let me do her hair once a week as she found it difficult to go to the salon. I spoiled her as much as I could. My mother loved me and I loved her. Even though we had suffered a huge blow to our relationship, I never stopped speaking to her or walked away from her. Sometimes it seemed we could go from zero to heated in no time, but it never lasted more than a day. Mom always said we weren't supposed to let the sun go down with you still angry, which is Biblical. So even if it was a quick phone call to at least say goodnight, that's what we did. I tried to honor my mother, the rest I left up to God. I did not have a grandma on her side so I did not have an example of how to treat your mother. That could explain a lot about my mother, losing her mother so young.

I had learned a lot about my mom while Uncle Fred was on vacation. We would continue to discover more and more about mom's new condition.

Uncle Fred Returns

Well we made it through the two weeks, but she was not happy about having me there. She complained almost the whole time that she could take care of herself. Mother was never a person to say please and thank you. She was a very hard person to wait on. I felt taken for granted but I told myself, that's Maria, the Queen Bee. She had such a sad childhood story with her stepmothers. And as a result of being mistreated, when she grew up and was in control of her own life, she made sure she would never be mistreated again.

My mother was very demanding and controlling. She didn't wait and let me offer to do things for her, she would tell me what to do. Even though I was over 50 years old, I felt like I was a kid again getting ordered around. I thought my mother was just being mean to me, but there was so much more going on in her head we just didn't know. It was a whirlwind of emotions staying with my mother for those two weeks. I really didn't see the bigger problem we were facing at that time. When Uncle Fred got home I was so happy to get back to my husband and my home. But I felt bad for Uncle Fred.

Paranoia

Since my father's death, I became my mother's power of attorney and was responsible for all her legal and financial affairs. The next very painful burden to come from this task and her dementia was the paranoia. She started accusing me of stealing her money.

My father left her a comfortable amount of money and a good pension so she did not have to worry about anything. It was not by any means a huge sum. At first when I took over, I would show her the statements and figures and what I paid out for her. She had a pretty good understanding of her account as her expenses were the same every month, so not too much changed.

As time went on, she started to get confused and she would not remember when she had given someone money or the balance had changed. The more she forgot, the more I got accused of taking the money. My natural instinct was to defend myself, which resulted in an argument. I was offended and hurt that she would think so poorly of me when all I was trying to do is take care of her. I felt unappreciated and just plain sad.

Things began to really change. I really started to see a difference in her behavior towards me but I always tried to explain it, make sense of it. I thought, Well, sure she is getting older. When the elderly lose their independence, well it's very hard for them.

Uncle Fred was starting to have more and more trouble with her too. She didn't want to cooperate with him either. He was starting to become a prisoner to the house because if he tried to go outside she would scream for him to come back in. He loved to be outside working with plants and the yard but she was so paranoid about him falling and getting hurt, he couldn't stay outside for even ten minutes. She worried he would have a heart attack while he was outside alone and no one would hear him. Her worrying became excessive. It started to get on his nerves--it actually drove him crazy. Every day, this battle to be able to go outside was wearing him down.

My Brother's Death

My oldest brother committed suicide not long after my dad's passing. He was a Viet-nam Veteran, a husband, a father and a much-cherished son. It was the day before his birthday that my sister-in-law found him dead in their apartment. We were all devastated and shocked. I thought this news was going to kill my mother. She adored him. As a Mexican American mother, her love for the oldest son was almost adoration. She was very proud of him and in denial of his issues. He returned from the war with an excessive drinking problem. When he first returned, the alcohol abuse was not so evident. He seemed to handle his liquor pretty good. But as he got older he just couldn't handle it anymore. It consumed him.

When I called my mother and told her what he had done, that he had taken his own life, she did not react like I imagined. I thought she would be hysterical. It was quite the contrary. She was calm; she didn't cry out, she simply said, "Well, he did this to himself." She did not blame God, she did not get mad, and she did not lose it. Totally different than what I expected, knowing how much she loved my brother. I couldn't explain it. I just accepted it and in one way was glad that she seemed to handle the news of her oldest son dying so well. Later it would all make sense.

Incontinence

I called to check on my mother almost every day. One day, I could sense something was wrong in Uncle Fred's voice. I asked him what was wrong. He finally admitted to me that mother was having trouble making it to the bathroom. She was having accidents and she didn't want me to know. She asked him not to tell me. But the work became too much for him. Extra laundry and bedding as a result of this problem. He had bought her some urinary loss products, but they are not always enough. He finally told me.

I said, "Okay, what I will do is start coming every week to help more."

It took me about an hour and fifteen minutes to get to them. Again I blamed old age for this new problem. When I asked my mother if she was having trouble making it to the bathroom or if she had been having accidents, she denied it. She totally minimized the situation and said she had a few leaks. Until I spent the night again and saw for myself then she couldn't deny it anymore. We agreed to use the products available for incontinence. She did not want to use a diaper at that time. I agreed.

My cousin, Nurse Liz, told me that incontinence can be a sign of dementia. I did not know that. I thought all older people had trouble with their bladders, they just wear out. And it can be that. But when you have dementia, it can also be a signal from the brain that is not getting through to let you feel the urge to urinate. By the time she felt she had to go, it was too late. This is a very hard thing for an elderly person to experience. Mom felt like she was losing control of herself. She felt like she was becoming a child again. If she had an accident she felt so bad. I felt bad for her. She did not want to go out as much after that started happening. If she did, she didn't want to be gone for long or go far away.

I share this information because this is something people don't want to talk about. I never heard anyone talk about this. Had I known then that this problem, along with the other signs of behavioral change, were actually dementia she may have been able to start on a drug that slows down the progress of this disease. There is no cure yet. But I may have been able to get her some meds to help her mood swings and maybe for her to be a little happier. Nurse Liz told me once that whatever kind of person you were in your youth, dementia magnifies that personality ten times. Some get bossier and mean and some get to laughing at everything. I got the bossy/angry one. Oh Lord, I had no idea what I was in for.

Post-surgery Nightmare

My mother had several joint replacements. This particular time the surgery was her hip. She had always done well with surgery in the past. I never knew someone to have such a high tolerance for pain like she did. She would never take anything for pain after surgery but Tylenol.

Before surgery, the doctors offered a patch for anti-nausea from the anesthesia. I knew that we had never tried a patch before. He assured me that it was the latest thing and we should try it. So I accepted. When she came out of surgery she was groggy and appeared to be resting okay. I went home shortly after they moved her to her room and she was sleeping. I stayed in town at my sister-in-laws place so I could be close.

The next morning I got up early and went back to the hospital to check on her. She was awake and talking but very strange. She was seeing things that were not there and talking very confused. She kept asking me where she was. Others that came to see her noticed it as well. I had asked them not to give her pain meds just the Tylenol, so I knew it wasn't the meds causing this confusion in her.

As the evening progressed it got worse. She was not able to get out of bed unassisted but kept trying to do so. So they alarmed her bed. The nurses sent me home and told me not to worry they would take care of her to go home and get some sleep.

The next day it just seemed worse. The nurses told me that she had tried to get out of bed on her own and the alarm did not go off. She ended up falling on the floor just missing the sink. They found her and helped her back in bed and she had not hurt herself or her new surgery. She was still so confused and I was scared. It did not seem to be getting any better. That night when I left her and went to my sister-in-laws for the night I kept thinking about moms situation. What could it be? What had her so out of her mind. It dawned on me that the anesthesiologist had put the anti-nausea patch behind her ear and maybe they had not taken it off. I immediately called the nurse and told her about the patch. She hung up with me and quickly ran to check for the patch. Sure enough, it was still in place. It should have been removed right after surgery. They quickly removed it and we all thought we had figured out her problem, halleluiah!!

After a few more days passed she seemed to return slowly to her normal state of mind. She left the hospital and went to a rehabilitation center to heal. My mother was okay with this because she knew it was temporary and that I could not take care of her by myself. When we got to rehab she was still demonstrating some confusion and hostility towards me. She decided she did not want to stay there but we had talked about it and I told her I needed their help and she needed the physical therapy so she stayed but not happily. It took about a week for her to return to "her" normal state of mind. Then she became the smiley pleasant lady that she was before surgery.

Whew, was I relieved that period had passed. I wasn't sure she would return to normal and the thought of her staying in that confused state of mind made me cry. I felt so bad for her.

The Diagnosis

Soon after that surgery would come a full shoulder replacement, about one year later. She had developed a cyst on her shoulder that was caused by water collecting there due to the muscles around the shoulder pulling away from the bone. And this was very painful. The doctor said the only thing they could do for her to stop the constant pain she was in, was to replace the joint. I asked if a woman her age, mid-eighties now, could hold up for surgery. He said yes, she was in good health. They checked her heart and everything checked out okay, so I agreed to the surgery.

Of course because of what happened with the hip surgery and the anti-nausea patch, I requested that they not give it to her this time. The doctors said no problem. They went on and did the surgery. It went very well the doctor said! Oh I was so thankful to him and to God!! But when she woke up in recovery, the nightmare started again. She was totally confused and seeing things and wired. She did not sleep for the next two days. I had to stay all night with her because she kept trying to get out of bed. The nurse in the hospital couldn't stay with her all night, he had other patients.

That was the longest night ever. She kept trying to get out of bed and would scoot her legs over till they hung off the side of the bed. I would grab her feet and put them back in the bed. She would get so mad at me and tell me to stop hurting her. She would tell the nurse I was throwing her up the stairs over in the corner of the room. (There were no stairs in her hospital room). This went on all night long. Then she started seeing things that were not there. The same thing was happening like when she had been given the patch, only this time there was no patch.

The next morning the doctor came in to check her. I was still there and so I told him what happened all night and could he tell me why since she did not have the patch this time. Why was she hallucinating? At that very moment when he looked at my mother, he saw her talking to someone she said was in her bed. We could see there was no one in bed with her. The doctor looked at me and said, "Your mother has Dementia."

He explained to me that when someone who has dementia is given anesthesia it puts the illness into a fast forward speed.

Again we went to rehab for the recovery time. It took longer this time for the confusion to wear off, almost three weeks. Finally, she appeared to be normal again, only she didn't remember the surgery or the three weeks post-surgery. When we would talk about what happened and she couldn't remember, it would make her very angry. She thought I was lying.

I didn't know a lot about dementia, but my cousin, Nurse Liz. did. She would become my support during the rest of our journey with dementia. She was instrumental in helping me understand what the course of this disease is and what my mother was going through. I was so blessed to have a nurse so available to me. I realize not all people do, but I can share what I learned in the hopes that it will help someone else.

Every day I would go and visit my mother at the rehabilitation facility. She seemed to be mad at me all the time. She got mad because I did not want to leave her purse in the room. She could not watch it when she was sleeping and the facility does not want to be responsible for valuables. Maria did not want to let go of that purse!! I mean she was determined. I had never given my mother a reason to mistrust me with her things. She knew I had my own money. I had never taken anything from her so I did not understand why she was saying I would steal her money.

I would learn that this is common for a person with dementia. But at the time, I did not know this and it is very hurtful. To be accused of something that you are not doing or would ever do is so very hard to hear. It hurt even more when she would tell other people I might steal from her if I take the purse. Everyone knew me there and never questioned what my mother was saying and told me not to worry about it. But they can tell you not to worry, but I couldn't help it. The way they talk, they sound so convincing and they really believe what they are saying. My mother was becoming a stranger. As if she did not know me.

After two months in rehab she came home. This shoulder replacement was not as successful as the other shoulder she had done a few years prior. She could not move her arm enough to wash her hair or lift her arm to dress herself. It became more difficult for her to function on her own. More work for Uncle Fred.

We needed to do something.

Help Moves In

For the next year my daughter and her family moved in with my mother and Uncle Fred to help out. Uncle Fred was having trouble with his vision due to glaucoma and was unable to drive. So my daughter and her partner would do the grocery shopping and any errands. They also took over most of the meal preparation and the lawn care. However, they had full time jobs and were gone most of the day. There were issues that resulted from two families trying to blend naturally, and introducing a five year old brought its own challenges.

At this point, mother was still getting around her house all right because she had been there so many years and was familiar with it. She did not appear to be sick at times. My daughter didn't think she was sick at all. She saw mom's behavior as normal for her age, as I used to before she was diagnosed. I would learn later that the dementia manifests much more when they are removed from a familiar setting.

Although the company and extra help with the chores and cooking was nice, that still left weekends. They had their own lives and activities with their daughter and were gone quite a bit on the weekends. So, that still left Uncle Fred with mom all day, all week and still on the weekend. He still couldn't get away from her to go outside and work on the yard because she was becoming more and more possessive of him. She just wanted him to be next to her. She was still watching TV at this point, so that's all he did with her. The problem with that is once they were alone, she wouldn't stay watching TV. She would try to roam or go to her room and dig through a dresser.

She was a fall risk so Uncle Fred couldn't let her roam about by herself. He became her shadow. He was getting tired. I always asked him to let me know when it became too much and the time had come. He told me it was not working out like he thought and he was still spending too much time with Maria.

I said, "Don't worry, she is my responsibility and I appreciate all the years you stayed with her. Now, it's my turn."

I suggested that he and mom move in with my husband and me so I could take care of them. Traveling back and forth was also too much for me. I also did not want to leave my husband alone all the time because I was gone taking care of my mom.

They had been in that house for over 25 years. Oh my, the things we can collect in that amount of time! The move would require they sell the house and get rid of most of their belongings. My mother did not want to do this. She was not ready to give up her things or her home of so many years.

My daughter didn't think it was a good idea either. She wanted to stay and didn't feel things were that bad. Uncle Fred felt differently. I promised Uncle Fred when it became too much for him, just to say the word and I would step in. He did not feel he could go on with her in this condition. Everything was just pushing him to the edge. Along with mother's behavior changing and becoming clingy and bossy and irritable, Uncle Fred was not used to dealing with more people and their problems. He was just becoming more and more stressed. Two older adults are used to having their house and things in a certain order. They were very clean and organized. The house changed with a child and two more adults adding to the work in the house.

These new stressors on top of mom changing made up his mind. He agreed to sell the house and move in with me. It would have been very difficult to get mom out of there without him. Plus, since he couldn't drive anymore, it would be good for both of them to relax and let me help them. We told my daughter they were moving with my husband and me and they should look for another place. She did so reluctantly .

She was not convinced the doctors had diagnosed my mother correctly. It would become an issue between me and her.

With the help of Uncle Fred, we convinced mother it would be best for them to move with my husband and me. My mother did not understand about the dementia. My mistake was trying to explain it to her. She would say she did not feel anything was wrong with her.

By this time she could not even take a shower without help. She no longer could do simple daily tasks by herself. She had fallen several times in the three years before the move and only once had to go to the emergency room because she hit her head on a table trying to get her own coffee. I lived too far away to get there quickly so I had to rely on help from other family members.

My husband's brother and wife lived around the corner from my mom and Uncle Fred. My sister-in-law was able to go check on my mother after the fall where she hit her head. She reported that mom's head was bleeding a little so we decided she should go to the hospital. It turned out to be okay, she was not seriously hurt, but I didn't want to take any more chances of her falling and this happening again. I told her it was best they come live with me. She finally, reluctantly, agreed to move. Thank God for Uncle Fred decided to come too. He seemed so depressed with his life and I assured him once they were with me things would be different.

The Garage Sale

It was very hard for Maria to see her furniture and belongings go out of the house to the driveway for a garage sale. She had really nice furniture, old, but good quality. I felt so bad for her but I knew it had to be done. It was far too much polishing and cleaning to maintain that furniture and she could no longer do it. Asking Uncle Fred to do it was not fair. He already had all the other responsibilities of the house.

Needless to say, the furniture flew off the driveway. It was a very successful sale. The hardest thing to sell is clothes. My mother had every closet in the house full of clothes. What we were unable to sell I gave away. Some of her better clothes she did not want to part with I agreed to put in storage for her. That I can tell you was a waste of time and money. She never used any of it or even remembers what was in the storage. But it made me feel good to know I could produce it if she asked for something.

This sale took two days. It was not easy. My mother was so unhappy with me. I was the bad guy. Why were people listening to me and not her? It was tough for me to make these decisions. I felt I had no choice. Her primary caregiver was tired and could no longer tend to her. The thought of a nursing home at that time was not an option. I believed you take care of your parents when the time comes. She still had a lot of life in her and didn't seem that her illness was that bad to warrant a full-time facility. She still ate very well, had a healthy appetite and slept most of the night. So a nursing home did not seem to be the right fit at that time.

It was a huge undertaking to empty the house but we did it with much help from our family and friends. After you move all the "stuff" out then there is the job of cleaning the house. Uncle Fred was not able nor did he have the time to deep clean. And even my daughter did not have much time to help with cleaning because she worked. Thanks to my best friend and my sister-in-law who came over to help me clean and load the dumpster we placed in the driveway to throw away the trash, it was done. The house was empty and clean and ready to sell. Now they would move a few of their belongings and clothes in with us.

There was much work to do at our home to prepare for their arrival. We remodeled the basement to make an extra bedroom and bathroom and living space so my husband and I could move downstairs and leave mother the first floor. Uncle Fred was in good shape physically, so we gave him the upstairs bedroom and bath. They brought their own bedroom furniture so that was nice. We gave mom our master bedroom on the main level. It has a bathroom with a walk in shower. It was perfect for her as it is hard to get into a bathtub at her age. We fixed the room really nice with her things and power recliner. We were finally all settled in together and the next phase of our journey begins.

She's Not Happy

No matter what we did to try to make her feel welcome and let her know that this was now her home too, she was not happy. Every day she would complain that it was not her house. My husband tried to tell her we were happy she came with us so we could take care of her and see her every day. I prepared all the meals and tried to fix her favorite things. She ate very well and actually lost a little weight with me. I was not putting bowls of food in front of her like she would have Uncle Fred do when he was preparing the meals. I just served her a plate and she seemed fine with that. I also took her to her new doctor who I just loved. She was so nice to mom and very knowledgeable about dementia. The doctor was very surprised I wanted to take care of my mom knowing she had dementia. I told her it didn't seem that bad to me, I thought I could do it. She simply said okay. I was to bring her back to see her every three months.

I called Nurse Liz to discuss why mother was so miserable at my house she explained to me that change is super hard for a dementia patient. They feel unfamiliar with everything. They can't remember where things are and new memories are hard to form. For instance, every time my mother got up from the recliner in the living room to go to her bedroom, she would take off to the left, which was the kitchen. The bedroom was to the right. After months of being here, she still could not remember that. This caused her to be unhappy and this is what I was seeing.

When she was in her own home, the dementia was not as visible. She did not appear to have any severe memory problems or physical problems. Of course, most of the time we saw her sitting down or if she was moving about it wasn't for a long distance as her house was not very big. After the move to our house, the distance became much further for her to get from one room to the other. I thought it would be good for her to be able to walk more and get more exercise. Maybe that would make her stronger. She walked with a walker and quite bent over it. She was struggling to make it to the kitchen and then back to another room. She fell six times during her first year with us. It was getting harder and harder to pick her up. Her balance was off and it wouldn't take much for her to go down. I was starting to see the reality of her limitations now that I saw her 24/7.

The dementia was killing her brain cells a little every day the doctor said. It seemed that she declined quickly the second half of her first year with me. By the time I moved her in with me, Dad had been gone almost seven years. Her first symptoms, the odd behavior and the problems with the anesthesia started five years earlier. So truly mom had dementia onset for close to six years before she moved in with us. Although it seemed the decline came quick, in reality it did not. I was unaware of the onset. By the time the symptoms were severe, she had already been sick several years.

Every day brought new challenges. She did not want to use a wheel chair but I told her she should. I did not want to risk her falling and me not being able to get her up. One time I had to call the paramedics because I was alone with her. Uncle Fred was on one of his much-deserved vacations to Texas and I was the only one here with her. The paramedics will come and help you but if it becomes regular then they have to report it to the state agency for the elderly. They said then they investigate to see if the person is in the proper care for their ability.

We did start using the wheelchair and I felt she was safer in it but eventually she did lose more strength in her legs. It became very difficult to get her out of the house and into the car. One time on a doctor's visit we were walking out to the car, before the wheel chair, and she fell. The walker does not keep you from falling at all. I knew she was getting away from me and that she was going to fall, but I couldn't prevent it. Thank God there was a man sitting in his car in the parking lot and offered to help pick my mom up. I was so glad he was there. The wheelchair just made sense so I would not have an incident like that one again. My mother had her pride too, she did not want to use a wheelchair. I didn't think about all the things that go through their mind about giving up more and more independence. I told her the chair was just a safety precaution and that I knew she could walk. She accepted that and let me put her in a wheelchair.

With the wheelchair came more modifications in the home. Safety bars to hang on to in and out of the shower and bathroom. We had to remove anything on the floor that could cause her to trip from not picking up her feet if she was using the walker.

Later I was to learn that too was dementia. Shuffling your feet can sometimes indicate your brain is not getting the signal to the legs and feet to move. It is not only memory loss you see from dementia but many signals that the brain tries to relay but do not make a connection. How we walk, how we talk and how we think, it is all affected. Plus all the involuntary commands our brains are designed to do. For instance, blinking, feeling hunger or feeling full. Picking up our feet to talk, feeling the urge to use the bathroom and so on.

We installed an intercom and a camera so I could check on mom without running up the stairs or even when I was away from the house. This really helped my peace of mind. When I checked on her at night, and she was sleeping, I could go back to sleep until the next check. If she was not in her bed I knew she was on the move and I would come upstairs to help her. I was given a piece of advice not to move into the room of the person you are caring for. It comes across your mind to just stay with them so you don't have to keep getting up every two hours or whatever. But this is not good for them or for the caregiver. No one can watch someone else 24/7. So I chose to use the baby cam and it helped me to monitor activity in her room.

We also added a chair in the shower so she could sit down. My shower had a small four inch lip at the bottom where the doors are mounted. It was becoming more and more difficult for her to lift her foot over to get in the shower. She would hang on the safety rails but was afraid she would fall. So, I put another chair outside the shower, so she could sit, stand and step in to the shower to another chair. That worked pretty well for a while. You have to get creative and do what works for you!

To help her get into the car easier, we had a step made like a platform that we could place on the ground when we opened the door. She could step up on the platform and then into the car.

Even holding her coffee cup was becoming difficult, so I got her a plastic cup which was much lighter and she could hold it without shaking. We were adapting to our new Maria.

Don't get me wrong. Even with all these things in place to help accommodate my mother, it was grueling. It is very hard to care for someone day and night. Nurse Liz said to me, "Lety, she is going back to a time when she was a child." She told me she is unsteady on her legs like when you was a toddler learning how to walk. She has difficulty holding her fork and aiming for her mouth. She doesn't like going to bed alone in the dark. She was becoming my child and I was her mother. I started to talk to her like she was my child. I spoke sternly sometimes especially if she was doing something that could be unsafe for her to do. She didn't like being treated like she was a fragile. She always insisted she could do things on her own, but in reality, she couldn't. She was doing less and less on her own.

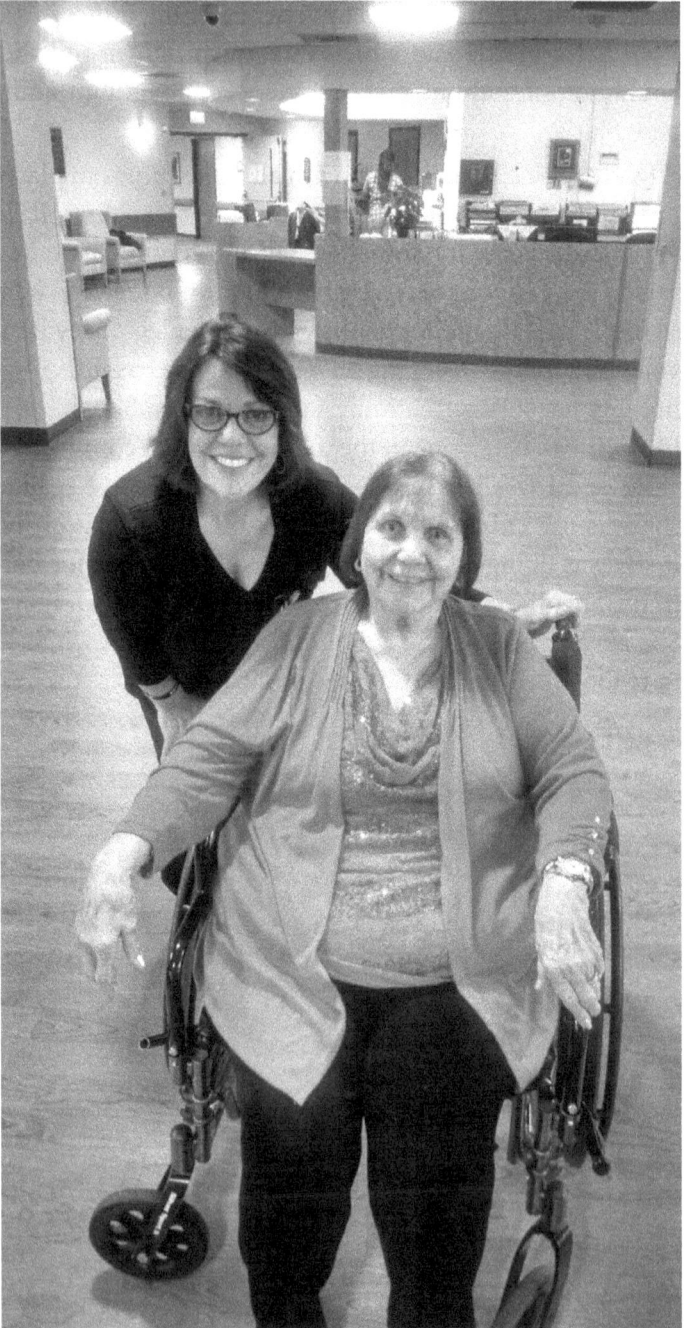

Sun Downing

My mother's behavior really took a turn after about six months of living with us. She stopped watching TV at night which is when she used to watch her favorite soap operas in Spanish, the tele Novelas. I thought she had lost interest because she couldn't remember the story line anymore. But something was happening.

Towards evening, when the sun goes down, she became very active. She would want to start digging around in her dresser drawers and opening and closing the drawers. She would take out make up and put it on at 9 30 at night. Harmless true enough, but then the arguments came out. Uncle Fred was tired by this time of night and he would tell mom to sit down and she would not. He would yell for me and tell me your mom will not sit down and I am afraid she is going to fall. She is not using her walker and just hanging on to the dresser. My mom would get so mad at him and call him a "chismoso" a tattletale or gossiper.

I would remind her what time it was and she should be getting ready to go to bed soon. She did not want to go to bed. She didn't understand why we all just didn't go to bed and leave her alone. She could take care of herself and she could go to the bathroom fine. Sometimes it would be closer to 11:00 p.m. before we could get her down for the night. Many times I would just tell Uncle Fred to go on to bed so he could watch TV in his room and I would stay with mom. She didn't want me though, she wanted him.

When she would get tired the confusion was worse. Arguing with me bought her a little more time with us so she wouldn't have to go to bed. She would complain and say I just wanted to put her to bed like she was a child. I would try to tell her, "No Mama, I just don't want you to fall and get hurt. Please go to bed."

I was tired at the end of the day. My day started at 6 am and after preparing three meals a day and all that goes with that and all the rest of the chores and not sleeping at night, I was tired!! Every day I asked God to forgive me if I was not being the best person I could be. It is awful to feel that you are failing in your God given purpose. If this is what I had to do in life, then I wanted to do it cheerfully. But I was not cheerful anymore. I was feeling bad most of the time. I was getting burned out. I was not able to honey her and baby her like she should be treated. I was too frustrated and tired most of the time. I had started smoking again after quitting for eight years. The stress was taking a toll on me, and I didn't want to admit it. There were days that she would wake up and seem normal. It seemed like she was okay and very clear headed. She would even tell me to have patience with her when she gave me a hard time. I wouldn't believe it. It was a wonderful moment of clarity when she seemed like her old self. I would think, It's going to be okay. I thought she was getting used to being here. But it was short lived. They were only pockets or episodes of clarity of a time in our past that would never be again.

Therapy

My daughters were concerned for me and advised me to seek therapy to help me cope with my stress and anxiety. My oldest daughter found a therapist online in my area and recommended I call her. My other daughter as well had used therapy herself and found it to be so helpful in her own healing with her own issues and wanted me to give therapy a try as well. I had tried going to therapy a couple of times in my life but did not have good success with it. You have to find the right person, the right fit or it can seem it is not helping.

I was open to trying again because I knew I needed help. And what a help she was! She was a godsend, a woman my own age who I clicked with. She actually listened and asked questions that made me think. She helped to explain why I was feeling a certain way. She enforced positive thinking and gave me tools to help myself when I faced high stress situations. She helped me to NOT feel guilty. I knew better being a Christian, that God did not want me to feel guilty, I was forgiven. Yet I felt guilty and bad every day that I failed at making my mother happy or just getting thru a day without an argument. I started seeing her about seven months after my mother moved in with us. Best thing I could have done.

The good thing about therapy is I had someone, a professional, to talk to and didn't have to worry my friends every day with my problems. My friends and family were great about letting me vent but you start to feel bad about burdening them. I couldn't take any more "bad" feelings. My therapist was so instrumental in me keeping my

sanity. I now had someone not only to vent to, but to help me understand what I was feeling and how to deal with those feelings.

The most important thing that came out of my therapy sessions was that I needed help with mother. I needed a sitter for an adult. I learned there are many agencies in place to help with caregiving. They will come to your home for a minimum of two hours a day. They accept private pay or sometimes Medicare will pay. So I tried a few of them, but it was hard to leave mom with a stranger. I knew I needed a break and time away from mom would allow me some time to recover. The first time I only left for two hours. It seemed to go all right. The problem is getting the same person to come back, you have to take whoever is available when you call, unless it is a standing appointment every week. That didn't work too well for me with a dementia patient because they can't be introduced to new people all the time; it is too confusing.

What ended up working for me was a private person who was recommended to me by someone in the business. She was a young gal starting out as an aide. She had just finished her course in caring for the elderly and was not yet employed by an agency. I gave her a call and she agreed to come out and meet mom.

She turned out to be perfect for mom. My mother liked her and she was great, her name was Ashley and I will never forget her. She listened to my mom's stories and watched westerns on TV with her. Mom loved her some John Wayne! She served mom her meals and cleaned up after her. One time when she came over mom had an accident and didn't make it to the bathroom and she put her in the shower and had her all cleaned up by the time I got back. She was totally competent and I had no worries when I left mother with her. We had a standing appointment every week so I knew I had a block of time for me. My therapist was right in suggesting I make time for myself, it is very important. Even if I didn't have anything in particular to do, I got out of the house and had me time. This is the best advice I can share with others.

Having Ashley to help was also beneficial to Uncle Fred. When Ashley came over to sit with mom, Uncle Fred could disappear and get some alone time for himself. Getting a break from listening to my mom was gold to him. This man had the most a tremendous amount of patience, but even he was starting to break down. He loved to go outside and mother just wanted him by her side. Ashley was a great relief to him because when she was there he could slip outside and tend his little garden. When Uncle Fred did slip away from her she noticed right away. Mother would tell Ashley to go find Fred and tell him to get back inside. She would try and distract her with questions about TV or if she wanted to do her makeup. But my mom thought Fred had been gone for hours when it was only ten minutes. She even had to wheel her to the window so she could see for herself that he was okay, even though once she saw him through the window she would start yelling at him like he could hear her to come back in the house. I started using Ashley for longer periods of time think that would be enough relief for us both, Uncle Fred and me, but it wasn't. It just wasn't. We were all getting so tired.

The Birthday Party

It was late summer and Mom's birthday was approaching. She would be turning 88 years young. I thought about giving her a party but then wondered if I should wait till her milestone birthday at 90. One of my daughters, who was visiting from California, suggested I just go ahead and do the party since she was here and could attend. Plus at her age, we didn't know if she would be blessed with 90 years.

It made sense, tomorrow is not promised so we should enjoy today. I told my daughter let's do it!! We all took part in planning mom's birthday party. We invited the whole family and close friends. We decorated and prepared lots of food and got a cake, it was really nice.

She seemed happy to see everyone. One of my daughters made her wear a birthday crown and funny glasses and she put them on and was a good sport about it, laughing and having a good time. She was actually quite a ham that day. I even have a video of her getting up from the wheel chair trying to dance with Uncle Fred and my granddaughter's father. She had a ball! She was hanging on tight to her dance partners! She couldn't move like she used to of course, but even one-stepping was dancing to her. We ate and had cake, sang happy birthday, she opened gifts and laughed a lot. It turned out to be a great party. The weather was perfect to be outside sunny but not too hot.

Everyone started to say good-bye as it was getting towards evening and it was over an hour drive home for them. My cousins, including Nurse Liz, were the last to leave. When we brought mother in the house something happened. She changed her demeanor and did not look happy. I asked her if she had a good time and she looked mad. I said what is the matter? Why don't we get you out of these clothes and put your night clothes on so you are more comfortable? She was not having it.

"NO, you leave me alone!" she yelled at me.

I was shocked. I said, "Mom what is it?" She was becoming more agitated and I didn't know why.

"Just leave me alone," she screamed. Nurse Liz stepped in and took over. I left the room. Nurse Liz said, "C'mon Tia (auntie) I will take you to your room and help you change."

She agreed to go to her room but did not want to change her clothes. After waiting on her to calm down she finally agreed to change. When I came back into the room my mother said to Liz, "There is the woman that takes care of us."

I looked at her with disbelief at what I heard her say. When Liz and I left the room she explained to me that she was sun downing, the confusion that sets in in the evening. They are fine one minute and then it hits so suddenly; the unrest, the confusion and the hyperactivity. You feel terrible when you see them like this. I felt so helpless.

I just wanted her to be happy with her day and it ended up so sad. My cousin Liz tried to tell me not to take it personally. Mom could not help it. I was the closest person to her and so I was the one she took out her frustration on. I was surprised to hear from the other family members that while the party seemed to be going so well and Mom looked so happy, she was complaining about me to them the whole time. It was very hard for me to hear this. Now looking back and realizing what dementia does to people, I understand. But when you are going through it in present time it is so difficult to make sense of reality for them. I cried so much during episodes like these. Her telling people I mistreated her or that I was taking her money hurt so bad. I was so glad Uncle Fred was my witness that none of that was going on.

I was so glad my daughter talked me into having that birthday party for her because it ended up being the last party she had.

The Medicine

I started to get really concerned when Mother didn't want to take her medicine. She would say I had already given her medicine and that I was trying to poison her. I explained she had not taken her meds for the day but she didn't believe me. Talk about frustration! Her answer was always just, "Leave it there and I will take it later."

My daughter suggested I use the Monday – Sunday pill boxes so she could see which day she was on. I would show her the container to show her that she had not taken the medicine for that day but that didn't work. I finally had to call the nurse at her doctor's office and tell them to please tell my mom to take her medicine and that it was ok to take all her pills at once in the morning as the doctor recommended. That made more sense than trying to have her take medicine at different times of the day. My mom would say okay to the nurse, but when she was off the phone she would get mad at me for "telling" on her.

In my frustration, I just said, "Fine, if you don't want to take your medicine, then you are the one who is going to get sick or possibly have a stroke. Is that what you want?"

Every day became more and more of a challenge just to get her to take her meds.

I wasn't able to get Mom to do the simple things in life she had to do. Taking her medicine, taking a shower, eating the food that was good for her and going to sleep at night were becoming impossible. I began to feel that I was failing as her caregiver and that I was failing God for not having the patience I needed to be nice while she was being stubborn. The truth was, no matter how good my intentions were, I was not trained to take care of a person with dementia.

Looking for Help

I decided to start researching the care facilities in my area. The first thing I learned is that there is a often a waiting list. You just don't decide to take them somewhere and admit them. Depending on weather you are private pay or you need help with the financing may determine how quickly you get a bed. There was actually a place I loved near my home and the wait was two years. Imagine you are at the end of your rope and you hear you have to wait two years! So I kept looking.

The first place I looked at was very big and seemed really nice. It was very clean and lots of staff. The lady showed me around the facility. The rooms all had two beds to a room. It didn't look much different than a hospital room. However, it was going to be a big change from the room I had my mother in at my home. The room only offers a small closet and nightstand for your personal belongings. I went ahead and placed her name on the list and continued to search out other care facilities. As I left there I remember crying and feeling awful. I called my daughter and told her I could not take care of mom anymore and that I realized my limitations and was looking to place Mom in a home. I didn't feel I had her support and that ultimately I was going to have to make this decision alone. My daughter never thought I should have taken her out of her own home to begin with. There are always family members that are in denial of a diagnosis of dementia. It may be as simple as them not being able to face the fact a loved one is slipping away into this illness. I really hoped she would understand where we were in this journey as her opinion mattered to me. In the end I realized I had to make another tough decision on my own.

I cried so much and missed my brothers, I wished I was not alone and they could help me with this decision. I did have Uncle Fred who felt the same way I did in that Mother could best be served in a full time care facility. His opinion mattered as he had provided so much of her care in the last eight years. Over the next six months I looked at several places as I watched my mother decline.

The Decline

Certain foods were not agreeing with Mom any more, like bananas. They made her have diarrhea. I quickly found out after being the one who fixed her meals. Naturally, I took them away. Bananas also are high in potassium, which was not good for her as she had too high potassium level any way. Lord, she loved her bananas and wanted them. I tried to explain the bananas were causing the diarrhea. I didn't want her to keep having accidents not being able to get to the bathroom quick enough. She did not understand nor believe me that they were the cause. All she remembered is she had always eaten bananas and they never made her sick. Actually, any fruit, grapes, strawberries and apples, all had the same effect on her digestive system.

Another thing she could no longer stomach was beef. My mom was a huge beef eater, she loved her steaks! Again, this would go right through her and cause accidents and I would have to put her directly into the shower. At these times she realized it must be what she was eating. Once she even apologized for being so much trouble. She even said just take me somewhere they can take care of me. I would tell her, "Mom, you are not too much trouble," but I was scared.

It was getting to be too much for me and I didn't feel she was getting the proper care. Her nights were getting so bad she would not sleep. She did stay in bed because I told her she had to let me get some sleep. But I don't think she actually slept. She was seeing too many things at night that weren't there. She thought something was crawling around in her room like a small animal. Other times she thought there was a hole in her bed and she was sinking. Another time she tore all the tassels off her pillowcase thinking they were spiders. I found a pile of them next to her in the bed in the morning. That explained why she was so tired during the day and napped after breakfast and lunch. She was always asleep in her recliner during the day. Nurse Liz told me to take her back to the doctor because once they start to decline it can come quickly. I took her advice and took her back to her doctor.

When we went to see the doctor, she asked Mother if she could bathe by on her own, Mom said no. She then asked her, can you prepare your own meals and again Mom said no. Next question was, can you dress yourself? Another no. The doctor asked her one more question, can you take care of your own house cleaning and laundry? The final no. She then asked her to do a simple cognitive test. She drew a clock on a piece of paper and told my mom to draw the hands in to show it was 11:00 o'clock. She was unable to. There were a few other things she wanted her to copy, and Mom couldn't. At this point the doctor told me my mother needed to be in a 24 hour facility. She told me no one person can care for someone else 24 hours a day and mainly because I was not qualified in handling dementia.

The average facility in my area cost about $7,000.00 a month. After you sign up on the waiting list to be admitted you just wait until they call when a bed is available. I put my mother on several lists since it was going to take time to hear from someone.

I was afraid of going through another winter with Mom because taking her out in her wheelchair to the doctor was so difficult. I actually felt scared trying to get her down the step of the door of my house to get her to the car. Then pushing the chair in the snow was almost impossible. I just had to find something before the winter.

I started looking at facilities outside my area, closer to where my mother used to live about 90 miles away. There was a chance I could get her in the same place she had done her rehabilitation after her surgeries. They knew her there and I loved the people there. Only problem is I would be an hour away and it would mean a lot of traveling for me to go visit her and advocate for her. Our need was so great; I decided it was worth it. After all, there were other family members who lived near that particular facility and they could visit, I thought. Especially my daughters who could help out if I couldn't make it into town, I thought. I added Mom's name to their list.

After not hearing from any other facility with a vacancy and another newer facility that was open and taking patients but not dementia patients, I accepted the first facility that could take her which was the one where she did her rehab. It took a couple of months from the time I put her on the list for the call that there was a bed available. They said they would do an intake evaluation to see where she would best fit in as there are different levels of needs. I couldn't believe the time was actually here and I was faced with this decision to leave her in this place.

When I got the call they were ready to receive her, reality set in. There were so many emotions for all of us. I thought of Uncle Fred and how much younger he was than mother but was living a life at her age and pace, and how tired he looked. I thought of my husband and how I had neglected him so much in order to have time to tend Mom. I too was so tired at night I just fell into bed. My husband never complained about my mom or Uncle Fred being with us he only showed concern about me not sleeping or getting enough rest. I thought of the quality of life mother had with me. She didn't want to dress; she stayed in a nightgown all day. She slept most of the day away. She couldn't talk on the phone any more with any one because she would forget to hold the phone to her mouth and people couldn't hear her. Most of her friends had passed already so we didn't get many visitors. I think meals were the only highlight of her day. She stopped going to church when my father died, so she had no social life. I prayed, please God, help me to do what is best for her. I loved my mother but just couldn't keep up with the demands of her illness. I had to make a decision. Thank God for Nurse Liz! She said to me, and I will never forget, "It is not a sin to place your loved one in a nursing home. It is a sin to forget them!" She witnessed many people who would leave a loved one in her facility and then never come to visit them or spend time with them. I made sure I would never do that to my mother.

Telling Mom It's Time to Go

Telling my mom the facility had called and a bed was available was hard, especially when it was sooner than I imagined it would be. I only had a couple of days to make up my mind. Many people needed and were waiting for a bed so they needed an answer quickly. There shouldn't have been anything to think about. I obviously needed the help. Yet I hesitated. My mother had become my child. I felt as though I was dropping a child off at an orphanage. It's funny how they say the cycle of life is to start as a baby, then a child then and adult and back to a child again. My mother looked at me in a different way than ever before. She even called me mother a couple of times. I would say, "Mom I am your daughter," and she would just smile and say, "I know."

I prayed for strength, which did come in my hour of need. God gave me the courage to admit I could no longer give my mother the care she needed and turn over the task to those who were better qualified than I. It had to be grace because I know I could not have been so courageous to make this decision.

I got Mother to agree to go willingly to what would become her new home by telling her it was the same place she did her rehabilitation. She did remember the place when I told her. And I told her they were going to help her get her strength back and get her legs working again. She thought it was her replacements not working correctly. So she agreed to go. Thank God. I did tell her if she became strong enough to walk by herself, she could come home. This time, she was placed on the long-term care side of the facility.

When we arrived, we were greeted by the admissions staff, wonderful people who are so understanding and compassionate. They were so anxious to make mother feel welcome. A few of the staff actually remembered Mom when she was in rehab and said how glad they were to see her again and they were going to be there to help her.

They brought us to her room and her new roommate. She didn't even seem to notice the size of the room and that it was much smaller than her room at my home. They did explain this was not permanent but it was first available and when something more adequate for her became open they would move her. This particular hall had some of the further advanced dementia patients and other illnesses. Mother didn't seem to notice this. A nurse and doctor come to the room to examine new patients, which is standard procedure. They check their entire body from head to toe. After the examination, Mom seemed fine and was talking quite a bit with the doctor. After the exam it was going to be time to eat lunch. It also was time for me to go. The staff reassured me that she would be okay. I knew in my heart I was doing the right thing yet I felt so bad when I left. I cried that night and didn't sleep much. I called to check on her and they said she was sleeping comfortably so I thanked them and I thanked God and I tried to close my eyes.

Here I was worried about the room being small and having a roommate but actually they don't end up spending that much time in their room other than to sleep. In the morning they get her out of bed. Help her to the bathroom and get cleaned up. They would help her dress, which is something she didn't do with me. I couldn't get her out of her nightgown. Now she would dress every morning. My mother always loved her clothes and had many clothes to sport. So this was fantastic to me that she wanted to dress up every day in matching tops and bottoms and even her socks. She got a reputation for being the sharpest dresser in the place! She always looked like she jumped out of a fashion magazine so I was so thrilled to see this again. Who knew? She liked seeing people again. She wanted to look nice and really cared about her looks again. When she was home with me she would say why get dressed who is going to see me?

Now there were lots of people who were going to see her, new acquaintances some men and some women. Something came alive in my mother that had been dormant.

It was her pride and her self-esteem. She once again wanted to look good and feel good in her clothes. So many of her clothes were just stored and now she was getting to use them. If you held up two garments and asked my mom which one she liked the best, she would always pick the designer label without knowing it was. She had a good eye and always dressed her and my dad to match or complement each other.

I remember Mom telling stories about how poor they were when she was a child that my grandma would make her a dress from the potato sack. Grandma would wash and iron it and sew it into a garment. I imagine that is why her clothes were so important to her and she took such good care of them and didn't want to give anything away. Some things she kept for so long they were dated but that didn't matter to her. She might need them someday so she saved everything.

You can only leave about 8-10 changes of clothes with them per week. I would take a new set every week so she could rotate her clothes and I would do her laundry. They do offer to do the laundry at the facility, but I chose to do hers because I knew how careful she was with her precious clothes.

I was amazed at how quickly she got into the routine of mornings, getting dressed and going to breakfast with the other residents. She was actually starting to put make up on after they combed her hair. I don't think my mother had tried to put lipstick on by herself in years and yet now she was blushing and lip sticking!! Oh what a smile that put on my face! The nurses and aides just lavished her with complements and told her how pretty she looked and she would smile from ear to ear!

When I walked into the dining room for breakfast to check on her she was at the table with three other ladies. She had her food and coffee that she ordered herself! When she saw me she said, "There is my daughter!" I had not heard those words in a while. I was the lady who took care of her, I was her mother, she even called me a name or two we won't mention but now, I was her daughter again! I loved it!!

Independence

One of the things I failed to realize when I decided to place her in the "home" is that she was actually going to feel more independent. You think of a care facility as a place where they do everything for you. But in reality, what they offer are choices. Yes they do what you can no longer do for yourself, but they offer you choices every day. What do you want to eat? You get to pick from a menu. What do you want to wear? You pick out your clothes. What activities do you want to attend, when do you want to sleep? These are just a few of the decisions that were safely in her hands to make and offered her some control of her life again, some normalcy and independence. She thought she was living in her own apartment and when I would come to visit her she would dismiss me! It was charming! I loved it. Like especially in front of others, she would say, "Okay, I am fine you can go now." I would say, "All right, I will be back on Thursday," and she would say, "Yes, yes you can go now," like she was a big girl!

My little girl, who was once my mother, was telling me she was okay and I worried too much! My mother, in her dementia, was where I felt weak and defenseless like a child. It is what made me worry so much about leaving her with "strangers". Would they take care of my precious little girl? It was so scary for me at the time, and yet now only a short while into her new life, she is telling me, she is okay, you don't have to make a fuss over me, you can go!! Wow!!

I think that when I brought her to live with me, I smothered her with my good intentions. I had taken away what little control she had left of her life. But again I have to thank Nurse Liz, and will continue to thank her through this book, for bringing to my attention that Mom could sense she was losing control of her life and become angry and or depressed. It was the dementia. It wasn't that she didn't want me to do for her. It was brought on by what she could no longer do.

For instance, my mother was Mrs. Clean. I could never hold a candle to her standard of clean. I am the clean-but-lived-in look, and Mom was photo-shoot-ready for Better Homes and Gardens!! When she lived with me and saw me cleaning she would get so upset. I didn't know why until I learned that she felt useless. She felt she should be doing something. I should have been more sensitive to that and instead it looked to her like I was doing what she could no longer do. I would try and tell her, "Mom its okay, you cleaned and worked so hard for many years, let me do it now," but she could never accept that. But now that she was on her own she was feeling that independence again. She was a brave soldier, not afraid to be in her new home.

Sure there were good and bad days, but mostly good. The aides said she was getting used to the routine very good. The nurses loved her. She was telling them funny stories and making them laugh and she was the center of attention where she liked to be. I never would have believed the woman asleep in the chair all day was now on a schedule with activities and making new friends.

I could not give her all that in my home. Independence was so contrary to what I thought would happen by placing her in a "home". But they gave her a feeling of control of her life and making her own decisions and she seemed happier than she had been in a long time. For that I will always be grateful she had that period of awakening.

The Partial

One of the first things I forgot to tell Moms' aides is that she had a partial in her mouth. Normally, it is on their checklist. For some reason, it was overlooked on both our parts. Mom was always used to taking it out at night but I think because of the change of routine and taking her out of her familiar settings, she also forgot or didn't know where to put it. The partial stayed in too long and became embedded in her gum. When my daughter came to visit her she noticed she was talking a little funny and wasn't able to eat on that side of her mouth. So when my daughter checked her she found out the problem. The nurse immediately took it out and it was not serious thank God. There was a little bleeding but it did not hurt her. The doctor checked her the next day and there was no infection so it healed up fine. My daughter was upset and felt they were responsible. These things happen; it was no bad intention on their part, simply an oversight. I too forgot to tell them with so many things you have to do and papers you need to sign. My daughter became very vigilant after that incident. She never liked that her grandma was in there and this didn't make it any better.

It was an isolated incident and we never had any others after that.

The other thing a dementia patient doesn't need is a phone. They don't really realize what time it is and can call at all hours. Sometimes they forget who they have called or how often. They can't often remember where they left the phone, which I can hardly remember where my phone is either, so I decided against the phone. She wasn't talking on the phone at my house anymore anyway so when she asked I said I was working on it. She complained to my daughter that she didn't have a phone so my daughter got her a cell phone.

I didn't say anything because I felt a strain in our relationship already so I just let her have it. My daughter did not consult me about it. She was never really able to handle it by herself. She called a few numbers by accident mostly, like when she called my son at work. I know she complained to me that she did not know how to use it and I was afraid it would get lost. She left it on the dining room table once and I saw it and brought it to her. She lost interest in it real fast just like the staff said she would.

I felt bad that my daughter and I were not on the same page about Mom. I went to visit during the day and she went at night, which is when the sun downing happens and when mother would be in her confused or complaining state. So my daughter did not get to see her in the daytime like I did in her activities and having fun playing games or socializing. I needed her to be my right hand and to help me when I couldn't be there.

Our next issue of difference, my daughter and I, was bringing Mom food. Because the food is much blander than what mom was used to eating, my daughter would bring her Mexican food. Because of the changes in her system like I described earlier, she could no longer eat everything she used to eat. The outside food gave her stomach problems. Plus she would eat in her room instead of dining with the others. I didn't like her eating in her room. She came to look for her dining partners at her table. But again, I did not say anything to my daughter about it. Eventually the nurses said something to her about how the effect the food was having on her. Part of it was a medicine that she was taking that gave her problems with digestion. I just could not communicate with this daughter without feeling like someone was looking over my shoulder criticizing my every move and criticizing the facility.

This would eventually drive a wedge between us and I was left with no option but to put someone else as my second contact. I needed someone who would speak to me. I needed to be able to communicate. Things were just to strained so I asked my sister-in-law to step in because I had to go to California for the birth of my grandchild and knew that she would call me if anything came up that merited my attention. Mom was my responsibility. Mine alone. I had no siblings to share with and I didn't feel like answering to my daughter about what she thought I should do. In fact I remember telling her, when I am old you can have at me, but this is my mom and I will make the decisions regarding her care.

The trip to California was a much-needed break for me. I never could have gone if Mom wasn't in the facility. I left with no worries; I knew she had fresh aides every eight hours and doctors everyday if she needed one. I truly was at peace knowing she was in a good place. I knew my daughter would visit and check on her too. I appreciated her for what she did for my mom, but really that was between her and her grandma. Family isn't always going to agree. I am sorry we had our differences because a situation like this is stressful enough. She loved her grandma and my mother used her to complain about me. I don't think my daughter really understood how bad Mom's dementia really was until my mother told her that she thought I had robbed a bank because I had a new car.

I wish my daughter would have seen that when my mother complained about me and how I treated her, that it was the dementia and not the truth.

Many other family members were able to visit my mother as well. My nieces and sister-in-law went to see her. A good friend of hers also came regularly. And my cousins and my mother's nephew and godson also came. For that I was grateful that she was back closer to her old home. Had I kept her away, chances are they would not have been able to visit so far away. She was happy to get visitors, even though most of them got an earful about me! Sometimes it was good, sometimes it wasn't, but at least she was talking and visiting.

Thanksgiving

In October at the "home" they offer the residents a ride on their beautiful bus to go see the colors of the fall trees change. In Michigan, that is a beautiful time when the leaves turn golden and red and brown. I went with my mom on the ride and we had a ball. She was the life of the party. She kept telling the people to make the sign of the cross, (she was a good Catholic) and pray that the gal driving the bus didn't crash!! Oh they all laughed and the young gal driving was such a good sport! We had fun and after about an hour we came back to the facility. Mom really enjoyed it. I thought it was great that they had so many activities and outings for the residents who were able to be mobile, it was great.

November now, and it was Thanksgiving. I had always had Thanksgiving at my house and cooked for my mother and father so she would not have to. I had been married for many years, and so Mom had not prepared a Thanksgiving dinner in a long time. This was going to be the first year I did not cook at home because I wanted to eat with Mom at the home. They offered an excellent turkey dinner to family members and friends who wanted to eat with their loved ones.

The dining area was beautiful with white linen tablecloths and fine glasses and real plates! For a small cost to the guest it was well worth it. They set up the dinner in a larger room, not the regular dining room for the residents. I was so excited to dress Mom up fancy and wheeled her down to the special dining area for those partaking in the special holiday dinner. My mother however, did not seem happy at all. Why wasn't I taking her to the (regular) dining room? This was not the right room or her table. I said, "Yes mom I know, but today is Thanksgiving and Uncle Fred and I came to eat with you and there is not enough room for us at your regular table." I showed her where our name was on the table, reserved for us. She said oh, and stayed but reluctantly. You never know how a dementia patient is going to respond to something, but one thing I know for sure, change is not easy, it is not good.

The Move

After my mom had been in her room at the home for a few months, they were going to move her to another hall. The first room was temporary until another room more suited for her opened. That wasn't a bad move because she had not been there very long. But after getting used to that room, which takes a couple of months, it was time to make one more final move. This was the hall they believed was the best fir for her. The patients were a little more independent and lively and could talk with her. We all thought it would be a good move for her. I was a little worried about her becoming disoriented but thought with time she will get use to the new room. We loved her nurses and her aides in her old room.

They were wonderful to her and she liked them too. My daughter wanted her moved so badly because the patients in her hall were in final stages of life and it was hard to see. Most could not talk and often you saw them just sitting in a chair or sleep. Some look very weak. But truly, my mom didn't see what we saw.

She saw a lady that sat at a little table with her dolls. My mother would speak to her but the lady never responded.

One day, my mother asked me to bring her a doll so she could give it to her. When I brought the doll Mom gave it to the lady and told her, "This is for you!" And that old woman, who never said anything to Mom, lifted her eyes and looked and Mom and smiled.

When the news came that a room was open on a "better" hall, we quickly moved mom. I thought this was going to be great and that my daughter would approve and we could be happy for mother. The move turned out to be very hard on mom. It was very difficult for her to adjust. The dementia was progressing and change was so difficult for her. She didn't know where she was and didn't recognize the staff. I prayed with time she would make the adjustment. To make matters worse, they were remodeling so there was a lot of construction going on.

The move to the new room also brought a new roommate who was a spitfire of a little old lady! When I came into my mom's room and my mother tried to introduce me to her, and say, "This is my daughter" her roommate replied, "Who cares!" I just laughed to myself; she was a cute little lady. Her bark was worse than her bite! Mom always had a little fight in her so I thought she will be okay and eventually won her new roomie over.

It was December and it was cold and starting to snow. I was so thankful she was in this facility as I would not have been able to transport her to the doctor's office in a wheelchair in cold icy weather. For that I was grateful. The doctors come to them in the facility.

One day they wanted to take some of the residents for an outing with the passenger bus to see the Christmas lights in the neighborhood. I thought that was a great idea, after all, she really enjoyed seeing the colors tour in the fall. I was unable to stay to go on the ride with her, but decided she should be okay on the bus with the six other residents. Not everyone could go and I was happy they asked my mom so I let her go by herself. I bundled her up with her hat and scarf and gloves. Her first field trip alone I thought!

What a mistake that was! When she came back she was totally disoriented. She did not know where they had taken her. She did not know she was back at the home. She refused to take off her coat when they got her inside by the nurse's station. She wouldn't let them wheel her to her room. She kept saying this isn't my apartment. She did not recognize her new hall or that her room was down that hall. The nurse could not calm her down even after some time so they called me.

I had promised to watch my grandchildren at a school event. I had to leave and return to my mom's to get her to go to her room. Once I got there she seemed happy to recognize me and told me she did not know where she was. I wheeled her down the hall to her room and once she saw her room, she said, "Oh there is my apartment." It was the hall she did not recognize. What she remembered as her hall was where there were people sitting in the hall in their wheel chairs or the lady at the table with her dolls. She still had not retained the memory of the new hall, which was clear of people and equipment. Also the construction removed the windows to the rooms and replaced with walls for more privacy.

I got her changed and in bed and left. I always felt bad after this incident that I made her change rooms just because this hall looked better than the other. She didn't mind her other hall or the people over there. I could have spared her the confusion and discomfort of learning yet again more new surroundings. I just didn't realize how great change would affect my mother. Sorry Mom!

We were in our fourth month at the facility. Just one month into her new room. The nurses were just as nice there as her previous nurses and the aides too. I truly was happy with the staff and this care facility. You must really have a calling I believe to see this stage of life every day you come into work for eight hours. You come to know them, care for them and know that eventually you will lose them. They get yelled at, pulled on, complained about and yet they smile as they pass out the meds, clean up messes, wipe butts and take blood pressures and chart everything!! Whew! The pay couldn't be enough. To these angels of mercy, I will always be grateful.

Christmas

It's Christmas Season! The spirit is one of love and joy! Everyone seems a little happier. The decorations are up in the windows and there are Christmas trees adorned. Lights were shining bright!! I love this time of year! I went to see Mom one Thursday, which was my regular day of the week to visit. I found her complaining about taking a shower. Something really odd happened to Mom about taking a shower because all her life she was super clean and always took a shower, in fact she would even shower twice a day in the summer.

It had to have been the dementia that caused her to resist the shower. If I told her, "Mom, it has been a week since your last shower," that meant nothing. Time didn't really mean anything. She just didn't remember. I told the aide that I would take her to the shower and she would go with me. I ended up doing showers the last month to help the aides.

The biggest reason she liked me giving her a shower is she said they didn't scrub her hard enough to get her clean. She told me to scrub her hard! I teased her and said, "Mom, you like it rough!!" She would laugh and say,

"Turn the water on hotter!!" Once the shower was over she loved being clean and felt really good. She would let me dry and style her hair. She loved when I dressed her up and brought her out of the shower room and everyone said she looked so good! She started acting better and getting used to her new room. Things were looking up, I was glad, God heard my prayer!!

We had a meeting that month to discuss her care. Everyone involved in her care come to the meeting. Her nurse, the doctor, aides and a social worker. It is intended to give you a progress report on how they are doing and if their medicine needs to be adjusted or changed and to answer any questions you may have. One of the most important things on mom's file was a DNR. Do not resuscitate. My mother was 88 years young. In my mind at that age our life is in God's hands. Quality of life is more important to me than quantity of life. I did not want my mother alive but depending on life support or even drugs that keep your heart running but it is like you are brain dead. You are alive just because you are breathing not truly present in your own life is not quality of life. I had to make a tough choice about some medication she could take to lower her lab numbers, but would produce her to have violent diarrhea. That is not a life I would want for myself. But that day, her numbers were fine and her report was good.

The following week the little crotchety lady, moms' roomie, became ill. She did not come out of her room that day. It was the first time I ever saw her stay in bed. I had gone to the room to get Mom's sweater. When I saw her laying there I asked her if I could get her anything while I was there. She asked me to close the drape on the window, it was too bright. I said sure, and told her I hoped she felt better. That night, our cute little crotchety lady, died. When I came in the next day to visit Mom, her roomie was gone and another lady was moving in. I didn't know the lady that passed but for only a couple of weeks, but I felt bad for her and her family. It was our first death since Mom's arrival. Mom didn't really seem to understand when I told her what happened to her roomie. Or if she did, it didn't seem to affect her. The new lady coming in was very nice. Maybe she would like to talk more with Mother and that would be nice.

The construction was still going on during this time but nearly completed. It was looking very nice. The noise was back down to a minimum and Mom didn't seem to bothered with the workers and extra traffic anymore. In fact, she made friends with a couple of the guys and promised them burritos!!

My mom used to cook the best Mexican food and loved to gift people with her tamales and burritos. Only, since she wasn't cooking anymore, she volunteered me. So I made the burritos and brought them to her. That is her one gift she passed on to me they say, is her talent in the kitchen and her generous heart when it came to sharing that talent with others. She may have forgotten a lot of things by this stage of the game but not giving away food to those she favored. It brought people so much joy.

I asked her who she wanted to give the burritos to and she said, "No, let me pass them out otherwise they will like you and not me."

I laughed and said, "Mom everybody already loves you!! But c'mon I will take you around so you can pass them out."

She found her guys and lit up when they said thank you and even more when they came back and told her how good they were and how much they enjoyed them. It's funny what will stay in our memory. She had given away tamales every Christmas since I could remember to her close friends and doctors and family. I was happy she got to pass out food one more time.

There was one patient in particular she took a liking to. I will never forget how she found a gentleman that reminded her of my father. She said to me, "Look there is your dad!" He did favor him a little, but not really. He was much smaller. The poor man didn't know why my mom had taken such a liking to him and always wanted her chair next to his. She even would pat his knee if she was close enough. I think he started to get a little scared, like who is this lady! But he made Mom happy. Then she thought she had another boyfriend. I was just tickled. Mom was really having an awakening! She was funny. The belle of the ball!! Life was getting better with every day I thought. It's almost Christmas!

Christmas Eve

On Christmas Eve I went to see Mom and get her ready for the day. She took a shower, without protest, I did her hair and make-up and dressed her up real cute with some little white go-go boots. She loved her boots that went with her beautiful black and silver pantsuit and white sweater vest. She looked sharp! She was all set for Christmas Eve. Santa was passing out presents to the residents and Mom got a few too!! She didn't really get excited about gifts anymore. She just looked at them on the bed. We walked out into the dining and common area where the others were. She loved being out there. She wanted to know what was going on. They had a nice dinner that day and I left and told her I would see her in the morning.

Christmas morning, I dressed her up in another pretty outfit. This time, a pretty red blouse and different pair of boots. I combed her hair but SHE put her make-up on. She said she could do it! I said okay! I was so happy she wanted to do things for herself again. We went out to the dining room for breakfast. They had some really cool things planned for the day and she stayed out in the activity area. She rarely went back to her room before bedtime. She liked being social.

She had company for lunch that day, my cousin and a friend of hers joined us on Christmas. She was so fond of this woman because her grandmother was my grandfather's, on Mom's side, last wife, so they were shirt tail relatives. Anyway, the three of us had Christmas lunch with her.

I thought my mom was really enjoying us and I had to get up from the table to get her some creamer for her coffee. In that short absence, she managed to tell them that they didn't know me. That I had her there against her will and that I robbed a bank and they were not to believe me or she would never get out. Also, she told them that I was keeping her check. She never understood her money went to pay for her stay there.

I found out later of course that this is what she said. When I got back to the table with her cream, she said nothing more about what she had said while I was away. I felt so sad when I was told she said these things because how she must have suffered thinking those things. It hurts so much when you can't help them. There was nothing I could do but let it roll off my back and keep smiling.

After lunch her visitors left and I stayed till almost dinner and then I left too. I wished her a merry Christmas and kissed her on the forehead and went back to my daughter's so I could stay in town. I had Christmas at my husband's side of the family the next day after Christmas.

My husband was not with me because he had gone to Dallas with my son for a football game. Out son is a coach and we both wanted to go support him, but I wanted to stay with my mom.

When I woke up the next morning after Christmas, I told my daughter I wanted to go see Mom real quick.

She said, "Mom you just went the last couple of days, I thought we could go out to breakfast." I told her I just felt like I wanted to see her for breakfast since I was in town. I told her I would see her later at the Christmas gathering with my in-laws.

I got to the "home" and I found Mom at the breakfast table in her night gown. She had not dressed yet. I asked her why she was still in her robe; she had a blank look on her face and just said I didn't feel like getting dressed. She did not smile or look like her normal self. She said she didn't feel too good. I told her if she didn't want to be in the dining room she could go back to her room and have breakfast brought there. She liked that idea so I wheeled her back to her room.

Usually while the residents are at breakfast the orderlies change their beds. Mom got back too soon so it wasn't ready. I ran and got the sheets and made the bed and put her back to bed. I turned the TV on and her breakfast tray came and she was happy. She said, "Oh boy, this is better!" The only thing I noticed was that her voice was weak, almost gone. So I left and as I left I thought how nice it was to see Mom three days in a row!! I was happy she was going to have lazy day and stay and bed and get pampered.

As I was leaving the nurse was bringing a chest x-ray machine and said they wanted to check her lungs for pneumonia. I said, "Oh, I thought you had to be sick to catch pneumonia?" Mother had not been sick with a respiratory problem at all. Well they did say the x-ray was just a precaution. So I left.

Every time my phone rang I would check the caller ID to see if it was the care facility. I hoped that when they called everything would be all right and not be the dreaded "call" that would eventually come. Even the staff knows you get a little nervous when they call because they quickly reassure you when it is not an emergency so you don't panic. When the call finally did come through they did tell me mother had pneumonia and they were going to start her on an antibiotic.

I was surprised since she demonstrated no symptoms. No cough, no trouble breathing or anything like that. I was just glad they caught it early I thought and nipped it in the bud. I still called nurse Liz and asked her if you could die from pneumonia, and she said yes especially at my mom's age. But Mom wasn't sick like that, she would be all right. The nurse told me they would keep a close eye on her. I thanked her, and I put Mom in God's hands. I went on to my doctor's appointment and ran some errands. I had no control over that situation and I was trying to learn to just put it in God's hands and not worry.

Later that day, around five o'clock, I went on to my sister-n-laws for our Christmas. She always has lots of food and drinks to celebrate. I normally love to partake but that day I had one drink but for some reason didn't feel like any more. I don't think I ate either. I watched the kids open their presents and as soon as they were done, I decided to take my grandson home to my daughter's. She was getting ready to leave too, but he wanted to ride with me. I drove over to her house and dropped him off and told her I would be back I was going to the store. I had started smoking again after quitting for eight years. So I pulled out of the driveway and almost made it to the gas station when I got The Call.

The Call

My phone rang. It was the "home.". My mother's nurse was on the line and she did not say this is not an emergency! This time she said, "Your mother has taken a turn for the worse I think you better come in."

This was it.

The call I had dreaded.

The one I did not think would come for a long time.

Suddenly, it was here. I told her I was on my way. I didn't even pull into the service station; I just raced to the highway entrance. I was only eleven minutes away from the facility; thank God I had stayed in town and had not gone home.

The first person I called was my oldest daughter to tell her to meet me there if she could. But I got no answer. Because we were not on speaking terms I called and asked nurse Liz to call her in case she didn't want to pick up because it was me. My cousin called her and she did pick up for her. Liz told her to get to the home. I had no time to call anyone else. I just raced to the emergency nighttime entrance. As I was pulling up, the nurse called back a second time. This time with urgency. When I answered she just said "Hurry!" I said I am outside!!

I ran to the door and her nurse was waiting for me. I could see the worry on her face. She let me in, we did not exchange words, I simply ran. I ran to Mom's hall and then to the end of the hall where her room was. I don't remember seeing any other doors, just her door. I ran inside and dropped my purse and ran to her bedside.

Her eyes were open but in a daze. It was as if she was staring at something. Her breathing was shallow; I couldn't even tell if she was still breathing. I put my hands on her face which was still very warm and I said, "Mom, I am here, it's okay !" She did not respond, but instead took her last breath. It happened so fast.

The nurses were there with me and one of them stepped forward to listen to her heart and check her pulse. She stepped back and looked at me with tears in her eyes and said, "She's gone." She quickly told me that the hearing was the last to go and that she was certain my mother knew I was there. I looked at my mom and threw myself on her chest and hugged her and I cried. With tears in my eyes I asked her and God to forgive me if I failed her and I told her I loved her one last time.

I had been praying for God's mercy on her and to not let her suffer in that terrible illness. I hated seeing her in that confused state of mind. I hated the way she looked at me sometimes with contempt and she would say I looked at her that way too. I hated that she thought I had made up her condition and lied to get her in a home so I wouldn't have to keep her. I hated she told people I hurt her. I hated she thought I stole her money. I hated that she never really knew how much I loved her.

All the things that she had just said about me the day before were still fresh in my mind. The things she had told my cousin and her friend. I hate she died thinking those things. I was her only daughter and only living relative. I was all she had in the world. And to think I would ever hurt her was the hardest thing I ever had to go through.

How I wish I had my brothers to lean on, but God answered my prayer that day and took mother home to suffer no more.

When I thought of all the things my mother saw at night in her room, the animals, the huge hole in her bed and even in the care facility when she would call me and tell me there were people breaking into her room and she had to be quiet when she first arrived and did not recognize the nurse that would come in at night to check on them. The time she saw my father in her room at night and called for them to bring him a bed. When she couldn't discern what was real and what wasn't. When I thought of all these things that tormented her, I felt so bad I could do nothing for her. When you can't do anything else you pray.

I believe that God in his infinite wisdom chose to call my mother home so she would suffer no longer. I will always be grateful that she did not linger, or suffer long. I am happy for her that she too believed in the same God that I do and He did not fail her ever. Even if I felt I should have done more, I know all things work out for the good when you believe.

God does not want me to feel guilt. He came so that we could have life free from guilt and condemnation. He wants us to feel His love and have hope and surrender to him. And that is what I chose to do. I surrendered my mother to Him and placed her in His loving arms to continue the next part of her journey which is eternal life. One day I know we will see each other again.

Thank you God for giving me the strength to walk this narrow road me and my family had to travel.

It is my hope that my story will encourage others on the path to never give up when it seems like you cannot go on. And to not be afraid to reach out to the people that are in place to help you with your burden. A burden shared is less a burden. Don't be reluctant to reach out to the people who are trained in the care of dementia patients. And please do your research of your skilled care facilities and use one if you need to. It is good for both patient and caregiver.

And last but not least, know that you are not alone in your struggle. Reach out to people who understand, like a therapist or support group. They will listen and help you with the important decisions you face.

Life after Mom

After the beautiful celebration of her life attended by so many friends and family, I realized my work was done. Death is a part of life and I chose to share the wonderful memories and pictures of her life. The outpouring of love during that time was amazing. We will never forget Maria.

I was able to move forward with my life with my husband and children and grandchildren. After taking care of and losing every member of my immediate family, it did seem a little strange. I wasn't sure who I was if I wasn't taking care of someone. I found myself in writing. It was good to share with others in the hopes of reaching out and helping someone else who is going through where I have been.

God was there for me and He will be there for you. Invite Him, He will come. I ask that God bless the person reading this book and help them with whatever they are going through and give them peace in Jesus' name. Amen.

P. S. Uncle Fred found love after mom. He went to Texas to be with his brothers and family and met a wonderful woman who would become his wife. They were recently married and are very happy! A first marriage for him at the young age of 78. There is always hope!

I would like to make a special mention to the **Ingham County Medical Care Facility** in Okemos, Michigan. To all of you from admitting to the doctors, nurses and aides and even the chefs who prepared the wonderful meals, I cannot thank you enough for your help, understanding and compassion.

I would like to dedicate this book to my husband, Fred Walker, for all your love and support

About the Author

I am a sixty year-old retired mother of four. I have been married for over 30 years I worked full time for 34 years while raising four children from two different marriages. Life was very demanding and busy to say the least. I never in my wildest dreams thought I would be writing a book someday. But yet here I am.

My path took me down the road of dementia with my mother. You must learn along the way. Every day is new and a challenge. My story is simply one of hope and love. My faith in God gave me the hope to rise each day and face the good with the bad and love brought me through it. He can do the same for you. You are not alone. Not only did God help me with my mother, but also with my entire family.

My brothers have both passed and my father too. Our family battled AIDS and Suicide and Kidney Failure. Those were very tough battles I know I would not be standing without God's divine intervention. I thank Him for all those He placed in my path to help me, support me and encourage me.

In my busy youth, I never really had a dream. I just worked and raised kids and took care of a husband, battled depression, went through two divorces and lost my footing. I was not serving God then, and when I couldn't fight anymore, I surrendered my heart to the Lord and He put my feet back on solid ground. I believe we can do all things in Christ Jesus if He is Lord of our life. He has never failed me. His promises are true.

God put a dream in my heart. He put a song of praise on my lips; and joy in my heart again. I would love to share with others my story down this road of dementia with my mother in the hopes that it will inspire and encourage others on this same path.

* 9 7 8 0 9 9 8 8 0 4 8 0 4 *